WHITE DARKNESS

WHITE DARKNESS

POETIC TALES OF THE SCHIZOPHRENIC EXPERIENCE

SUSAN WOJNAR

First Edition 2023
ISBN: 979-8-218-26239-6

Pubished by The 7 Muses
30 Roslyn Drive
Youngstown, Ohio 44505
music4enrichment@gmail.com
www.susanwojnar.com

Cover design by Aaron Yozwick
Book design by Meredith Pangrace

For Skylar

Please, Please forgive yourself
—James Hetfield of Metallica

Table of Contents

Preface

Marauders

Silently
Slipping
Through bars in the window
Drifting
In a row
Miniature shadow people
Crept 'round the walls
Like the old woman
In *The Yellow Wallpaper*

They were Marauders
Bringing me
A melting sorrow
I could not rise
From my bed

They finished
Creeping
Sat 'round the hearth
Eyeing me
Through the gloom
Stole up the chimney
While I wept

I threw a dime
Into the fireplace
To pay off
The Witches

Introduction

Family Affair

My family's voices
Are in my head
Mocking every thought, every action
Their voices
As real to me
As the sun in the sky
The grass on the ground

My family doesn't know what's wrong with me
They don't know about mental illness
Spiritual emergencies
Or the spirit possessions
West Africans call
The White Darkness
Neither do I
They know I am acting crazy
Hostile, avoiding them
But they do not know why
I don't tell them, because I think
They know what they are doing to me

I feel hated, used and confused
Outraged to be persecuted

They are hurt, angry, at wit's end
They think I am on drugs
We all feel
Betrayed

No one can break down the walls
Everyone lets go
And into the fire
I run

Sound Affects

The Voices
Enter and exit at will
I feel them move in
Rummage around
My ear canal
Twisting, turning
Knocking about
Like marbles
They barge in
Talk in short sardonic bursts
Monopolize my thoughts
With long monologues
I cannot
Click off or fast forward
I cannot
Tune them out, distract myself or ignore their demands
I cannot
Simply stop listening
I cannot

The Voices
Do not want me to think about what is happening
I try to figure it out. I try to *think!*
They tell me to stop
I am scaring the children
They shout at me

"You're hurting people!"
They tell me
I am in heaven
Where thoughts kill
So I struggle
To think of no one

The Voices
Speak from my stomach
Feet
Heart
I am polluted
The clock
Demands to know who my family is
The nature of my relationships
What connections do I have?
I shout at it
Over and over
"Leave me alone!"

The Voices
Come out of my mouth
When I sing
One voice
Like a siren
Makes the blood
Pound and pound
In my head

The voices are
In the music
A nightmare
Of hidden messages
Piano keys
Mock me
Guitar strings
Whisper

Relief comes with catatonia
Standing
Staring
Frozen
Hours
Of blessed silence

Out of the Woodwork

I could see them
When I pressed
My eye
To the knots
In the pine panelling

Pointed heads
Long necks
Bird-like delicacy
Part human
Part creature

They stared back
Little families
In little rooms
In the pine
If I stared too long
They would slam the door
In my face

The One

Silhouettes
Line the sidewalk
Red, blue,
Emerging, fading

There is a fleeting
Calm
An invisible
Gnarly hand
Grabs my neck
Boney fingers

Pete shouts at me
From high above the city
He narrates my plight
He Sees All
Knows All
Says I am
The One
I have the Keys
And Everything
Is happening
Because
Of me

I hurl my car keys
Across the university lawn
Don't want the power they wield
I circle our Lady of the Most Holy Rosary Church
Hoping to find a priest
To cast out the demons

Searchlights
Cut the nightscape
They are looking for me
I board a bus
At midnight
Last one out
Passengers
5 or 6
Then 7, 9, 15
Appear out of nowhere
The driver peers at me
"You can't get on this bus."

Wandering beyond the last streetlight
My left hand is suddenly
Grasped by another
I pull away from the phantom feeling
It pushes deeper into my pocket
Why don't I scream?

The hand
Turns me back
Toward the lights
Of the city

Landlady purchased it
After her husband's
Suicide
She sees therapy
In restoration
Fresh from an eviction
She grants me a second chance

Barry and I arrive at Michael's
After a concert at Wilbert's
I still get out a bit
Though mostly
I'm confined to my cold, dim apartment
Transfixed by other worlds
Barry regales me while we await
Omelettes and home fries
Out of his mouth flows a
Thick, white, milky…something
Glanc-ing around the diner
I I see the "No Smoking"
sign
No cigarette pack, lighter or ashtray
On our table
The airy substance rolls in and out
Of Barry's mouth
He is oblivious
Going on about gigs, concerts, gossip
En-tangled in his words, a voice —
You see the Holy Spirit

The moment passes.
The Holy Spirit
Vanishes
Maybe I imagined this
Maybe this happens *all the time*
Maybe I am just now noticing it
I fear it is forbidden to speak of
Like everything else
I see

I risk it
Blurt out to Barry
Tell him what I see
He never calls me
Again

Little Caesar

Enclave of
Shaker Heights
They do
Caesar's bidding
Attendants
Clerks
Staff

See
They entrain
Into slavery
Every move
Puppets
On Voodoo Strings

I step into White Darkness
With an inner scream
Legs yearn to run
Nowhere to go

Caesar owns nine McDonalds
A jazz lounge
Speaks in commands
One leg is prosthetic
From Vietnam
Deck of cards with him

Always
Shuffling

I apply for a job
As a waitress
In Caesar's bistro
Become his masseuse
Housecleaner
Mate
Remove leg
Clean apartment
Lie in bed
Feel the stump
See
Tibetan Demons
Leap to the fore
From black lacquered
Chairs
Faces and fangs
Blow through the room
In a Himalayan blizzard
Frozen now
Something
I cannot name

But I know how Caesar
Became Emperor
Of all the land

The Dance

Made the move from cocktail waitress
To stripper
After yet another night
Of no tips
At the Babylon
Skirt was short
Top was tight
Must have been
My personality

Can't pay rent
Resumes rejected
Interviews going nowhere
Filed for bankruptcy
Ads promise
$1,000.00 a week!
I am adrift
In loneliness
And wonder if I can…

So I practice
In my second story efficiency
In the tree tops
Strip to my underwear
Put on Stevie Wonder
Superstition

Kenny Wayne Shepherd
De Ja Voodoo
I whirl and dance
Through the night
Driven by the wilding

As server
At The Babylon
I watched the girls
Not impressed
They didn't dance
They gyrated
Shook
Humped the floor
Swung on the pole
But they didn't dance

I would dance
First audition
A strip joint in Rootstown
Out in the boonies
I own no stripper clothes
So utilize my best Victoria Secrets
The girls were aghast
At my lack of makeup
They gussied me up
"You got to SELL IT, honey
Take it up close to the edge of the stage

And SELL IT," the DJ urged
But I *danced*
And failed the audition

Went back to the Babylon
They were not so choosey
And I could start right away
I left empty handed
Night after night
The money makers
Were in the VIP rooms
Doing it
While I grew invincible
On stages
Paying homage to the Goddess
Power surged through my manic veins
Up my spine
Into my head
The other girls said they had to drink
Or do Oxy's
To get on the stage
Not me

Flitted from club to club
Maybe a stuffed garter belt
Was just over the horizon
Never mingled much with the other girls
They were stereotypical

Hard
Haters
Despised men
Used them mercilessly
Who is the victim
at Strip clubs?
I left them to the game
They left me to the dance

Until I landed
At the New Affair
Star developed a distaste for me
Dumped body gel
Into my clothes bag
Ruining every stitch
Threw my street clothes, shoes
Into the dumpster
Forcing me to drive home
At 4 in the morning
Barefoot, in a thong and bustier
Culminated in slashing my tires
Three times
I took the hint
Quit the club

At Dreamer's Cabaret
A high school English teacher
Taken with my Aphrodite impulses
Talked with me

Sat with me
Sent cards
Letters
Flowers
Asked about my well-being
An English Teacher
Another hapless misfit
At The Dance
Vessel

I am used
Helplessly whirling
A tarantella
While phantom hands
Reach up and out
of the White Darkness
Snatch my ankles
Pull down down
I leap leap
To avoid their clutches

I am used
Arms Tremble
Flap
Against my will
My call for help—
For answers—
Brings Bill, the Bible,

The Black Church
He prompts
"In the name of Jesus, leave,"
But my puppet arms flail on

I am used
Rippling, rhyming words
Gush out of me
Unbidden
All Mississippi-Delta-
Hoodoo-Mother-Tongue
I am the mouthpiece of
A mighty river
Pouring out

Invisible Partners
Dance with me
Promenade
Cakewalk
I feel
Phantom knees
Touch mine
Push pull
I am
Tangoed
Used again

I am used
I am Nothing
I am Everything
The Great Spider of Creation
Spins through me
Thrown to my knees
In adoration
Staggering to my feet
In agony

Therapists, Doctors
Murmur and prescribe
Voices from the Shadows
Whisper
"Who is this woman
Now our songs
Are sung
Through her?"

Vessel

I am used
Helplessly whirling
A tarantella
While phantom hands
Reach up and out
of the White Darkness
Snatch my ankles
Pull down down
I leap leap
To avoid their clutches

I am used
Arms Tremble
Flap
Against my will
My call for help—
For answers—
Brings Bill, the Bible,
The Black Church
He prompts
"In the name of Jesus, leave,"
But my puppet arms flail on

I am used
Rippling, rhyming words
Gush out of me

Unbidden
All Mississippi-Delta-
Hoodoo-Mother-Tongue
I am the mouthpiece of
A mighty river
Pouring out

Invisible Partners
Dance with me
Promenade
Cakewalk
I feel
Phantom knees
Touch mine
Push pull
I am
Tangoed
Used again

I am used
I am Nothing
I am Everything
The Great Spider of Creation
Spins through me
Thrown to my knees
In adoration
Staggering to my feet
In agony

Therapists, Doctors
Murmur and prescribe
Voices from the Shadows
Whisper
"Who is this woman
Now our songs
Are sung
Through her?"

Fair Trade

Body parts.
They deal in body parts.
The cashiers at the Get Go
Leer at me.
My electric blue eyes
Coveted.
I grab my cigarettes
And flee to the car.
I call my aunt
To come and stay with me
But she too wants my eyes.

Tony The Pimp

Chunky
Middle-aged body
Poured
Into black leather
With Gerri Curl sheen
Tony the Pimp
Checks me out
We drive his white Cadillac
With TV, heated seats
To The Lancer Bar
He sips Hennesy
I savor
Grand Marnier
The orange liqueur
I grew to love
In the jazz clubs
of New Orleans
Boney James
Plays
"After The Rain"
Nothing definite
Is asked
or said

Tony is
Kind?

Calm
Conservative
He takes me
To an all night
Jewish diner
On the West Side
The wait staff knows him
Everyone is agreeable
We sit by the window
And eye the cops
That are circling
The building
Routine check
at 3:00 a.m.

Tony works
On his Surf and Turf
I pick at a salad
He takes me back
to my apartment
On the East side
He leaves —
A blur of blackness
And dusk
Maybe Tony thinks
I'm undercover
Or sees
Trouble

In the unhinged mind
of a hapless would-be Ho
Straight outta Suburbia
Masters Degree
Idling on the wall
Nothing definite is asked
or said

I don't know
What to say
In my phone messages
To Tony
I don't know the code
"I'm ready to work…"
I do not hear from Tony
I am facing
An eviction
And another
Christmas
Alone
I leave one more message
He calls me
From his cell
In my driveway
I descend
Three flights of stairs
Let him in
Neighbor
Gives Tony's ride

The Eye
In the foyer
Tony hands me three
Hundred dollar bills
"For your rent"
Nothing further
Was ever asked
Or said

Twilight of the Ashes

Ashes, ashes, falling down
Out of a predawn sky
I am driving, driving
Out of necessity
The mother of invention keeps creating
Out of my mind
Ashes, ashes raining down
From a phantom steel mill sky

A graveyard-shift canopy
Is it Heaven....crack it open
Crematorium
Bursting with the gritty sooty dead
Out of necessity
The mother of invention keeps creating
Out of my mind
Ashes, ashes falling down

I am driving, driving
Frantically dialing and dialing the radio
Does anyone else know
About this explosion over Mayfield Heights?
I roll the window up, down, up, down
Is this acid rain? Will it burn my skin?
It does not!

I am driving, driving
Through the gritty, sooty ashes of the dead
On Mayfield Avenue at 3 a.m.
I am all alone
I am not!
 A black man walking along the side of the road—
Does *he* see the ashes?
Yes!
He looks up to the sky,
Reveling in heaven's exhaust
Encouraged,
Because he is a black man,
I pull over to the side of the road,
Stick my face out of the window
And reach with my tongue
Towards heaven

I am driving, driving
Dialing and dialing the radio
My son's voice tumbles out
Rips and reaches
From inside the old school rhythm and blues
To his three years AWOL mother
I scream at the radio, "Can you hear me?
I can hear you
You are on the radio!
And I can hear you!
It's your mother I think I am dying!"

My son's voice insinuates itself
Between Al Greene's shouts and moans
He sounds bored, uninterested
I am sobbing, sobbing,
 "Are you alive? Are you ok?
I can hear you on the radio."
His voice, a monotone,
Fades in and out
Through the polyrhythms
I strain to hear his words
He is distant,
I am sobbing, sobbing
My son's voice -- embedded in the airwaves
But we cannot connect
I am sobbing I love you I love you I love you
I think I am dying just remember I love you
No reply at all
Is anybody listening?
There's no reply at all

I feel the dead
Their ashes
Fill me

I Scream The Body Electric

My eyes
Are seared
Electric surges
Reach my brain
Send shock waves
Down my spine
Energy
Pain
Leaps out
From lamps
Wall sockets
Like laser beams

I am frying
Frying
Power tools
In league
Against me
Every hedge trimmer
Weed-whacker
Chainsaw
Mower
Attacks
Through walls
Sending lightning bolts

I am frying
frying
Microwaves
Sizzle
Within me
Pulling pulling
On my inflamed
Brain
I feel my cells
Crisp
Explode
This will kill me
If I don't step away
I am frying
Frying
The sun reaches my retinas
Hot pokers, needles
I drive 'round and 'round
How to escape the torture?
I am weakening
Weakening
Pull to the side of the road
Slump over the wheel

I am fried
Fried
Police find me,
Question

Put me in the squad car.
I pass out
Awaken to bare cinder-block walls
Of the locked ward

What Was

There were sweltering summer nights
Pre central air
Just me and Dad
On the front stoop
Watching fireflies
Waiting for the house to cool down
Before bed

There was a purple bike
With a sparkly banana seat
High rise handle bars
Riding up and down
Our dead end street
Hair streaming
In the wind
On the downhill run

There was that small jar
Of decadent Hellman's mayonnaise
In my grandmother's fridge
With which she made exotic baloney sandwiches
"Bring out the Hellman's and Bring out the Best"

There were trips to the drive-in
Pillows in tow
Falling asleep

Half-way through the show
Being carried from car to bed
There were trips to Canada
To D.C.
To Gettysburg
To the Ocean
To the mountains
To the forest

There were fishing trips
Bluegills and sunfish
Pint-size rod and reel
Red and white bobber
Minnows
(continue stanza)

Shiny and slippery
So much better
Than touching worms

There was the shade
Of the mock orange tree
Where I made clover chains
And dreamed
Planting the garden
Dad placing a dead fish in with the corn seed
Like the Indians
To fertilize the soil
There was Charlie the cat

My father cried
When he died

There were trips to town
To pay bills with my mother
Slipping the envelope into the
Payment deposit box on the side of the building
There were BLT sandwiches
At the Minuteman Restaurant

When our errands were through
There were neighborhood friends
We imagined ourselves
Teachers, store clerks,
Cowboys, Indians
Characters from Lost in Space
There were toy animals and dinosaurs and Barbies
Playing dress up with the box of clothes
My mother had saved
A skirt with big red roses
High heels and shawls

There was a wading pool in summer
Sleds in the Winter
Leaves to be jumped in the Fall
Handmade Easter dresses
In the Spring
Holding still while my mother
Hemmed and pinned

Holding still while my mother
Permed my hair
"You must suffer to be beautiful"
But tomboys never were

There was whirling and dancing
To my mother's classical music
On the hi-fi
Pleading for a piano
Of my own
So I could make
The sound of freedom
There were lessons and practice
And making up songs
Whirling and dancing
At the keys

There were three sisters
There was the awkward middle child
An older sister who was too distant
A younger one who was too spoiled
There was jealousy, antagonism
Teasing
Stay on your side of the car
There was camaraderie, companionship, love
There was a middle class family
With a stay at home mom
A father who worked three turns

At the mill
What could possibly go wrong?

Cuckoo's Nest

Admitted on a 302
"Danger to self or others"
Enraged
To be caged
By the third day
I figured
You gotta get with the program
To get out
Kept to myself
Everyone else
Seemed crazy
The girl who ended up
In four point restraints
Three times in one week
The boy who still found the means
To cut himself
The man who talked of
Nothing but conspiracies
The zombies
In their private apocalypse

Self-preservation
Kept me quiet
About the extent of my symptoms
To avoid the Thorazine shuffle

Saw the doctor once for 5 minutes
Diagnosis was never explained
Plan for recovery never mentioned
Nothing was offered
Except medication
I walked the barren halls to pass the time

Up and down
Up and down
The Conspiracy Man
Tagging after me
Trying to get me to see the light

Ask Alice

One pill
Makes me stupid
Helpless
Staring blankly at pages
And people
I fake my way
With remembered social niceties
But I am not there

One pill
Sends appetite into overdrive
Weight goes up and up
Against all efforts
My brain
Never receives the message
That I am full
I buy yet another set of clothes

Not enough of one
And I am a raw nerve
Caught in a swirl
Driven
'Round and 'round

Another
Heightens my plight
Visual terrors
Plastered to my eyes
The voices roaring me
Into submission

I must wait
Wait
'Til it wears off
'Til I see the doctor
Who will guess what is right
"Let's see what this does…"
I tinker with the cocktail
Desperate bartender
In search of the perfect mix
The only control I have
It goes on my record—
"Non compliant"

When I get the mix just right
I re-emerge
See light in my eye
Recognize my face
Personality returns

The balance may stay
Or be suddenly upset
I am a demon
Pale ghost
Vacant shell
Once again

Vacant shell
Once again.

Tinfoil Hat

I molded the aluminum
To my head
I am well enough to know
This was insane
Desperate enough
To try
It worked
A little
The voices dimmed
For awhile
But I cried
Knowing I had donned
A tinfoil hat

Smokephrenics

Our Lives
Up in Smoke
Our brains
Smoked
None may peer through
Rusty coffee cans
Centered in our midst
Filled to overflowing
To untrained eyes
Useless butts
But they are the fire of madness
Turned to ash

Toxic fumes of
Our Glue
Rise and fall
Languish in stagnant air
Through our poverty of thought
Or fevered grasping of
Private worlds
We think upon
And think upon

Hazy pacing marks the passing of the day
Nicotine, embalming fluid
Preserves us with our reason to live

Because surely the very next puff
Will restore us
Surely the very next drag
Will stop the whirligig of our minds
Or fill it with something
That resembles motivation
On the cusp of hope
Chained
Smoked

Holding Pattern

I am Alice down the rabbit hole
Grasping as I fall
Shattered
From inside
"All the kings horses
All the king's men…"
Couldn't.
So I must remember
To Re-Member
Like Isis in search of Osiris
When the onslaught comes
I force myself
To stay in this world
Where my mother, sister, son, friends
All reside
It has taken me
Fourteen years
To learn to hold on
I am prepared
I recite
Drown my oppressors
With all my might
"My name is Susan Wojnar
I grew up on 603 Barker Ave.
New Castle, Pennsylvania
My parents are Louis and Joanne Wojnar

Both my parents grew up on farms
I attended Union Elementary
Graduated from Youngstown State University
Have a son named Skylar
I recite the name of every friend and relative
From the past
Every neighbor
Every pet
Scan every item in the house
Stare at family photos
Recall what knives and forks are for
Bathe myself in ordinary substance
Till the attack subsides
And my sobs fade
And I lie exhausted
But tethered
Making the center
Hold

Acknowledgements

I would like to thank the Fallen City Writer's Group from Youngstown, OH for their support and encouragement. Their interest in the subject and invaluable critiques sustained me whenever the self-doubts crept in. Very big thanks to Bill Koch for his keen editing. Thanks to Meredith Pangrace for her outstanding guidance during the publishing phase and to Aaron Yozwick for his graphic art talents in designing the book's cover.

As a mental health worker, I see time and time again the tragedy of those who are ill and either have no family or whom their families' have abandoned. It rarely ends well. So very special thanks to my family, particularly my son Skylar Slavik and sister Carole Wojnar Peter for learning,understanding, for forgiving, for accepting and loving me.

About the Author

Susan Wojnar holds a MA in English from Youngstown State University and is employed as a social worker in the Behavioral Health arena. She is also a professional musician and has played her original music in the Northeast Ohio area for many years. She is very fond of cooking, gardening, books, writing, music, swimming, running, nature, the theatre, The Great Lakes, family time, and cats. She is definitely fond of cats.

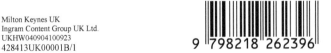